Comparison of fertility trends estimated alternatively from birth histories and own children

Robert D. Retherford
and Iqbal Alam

Number 94 · July 1985

PAPERS OF THE EAST-WEST POPULATION INSTITUTE

ROBERT D. RETHERFORD is Assistant Director for Graduate Study at the East-West Population Institute and Affiliate Graduate Faculty in Sociology at the University of Hawaii. IQBAL ALAM is with the Population Division, Economic and Social Commission for Asia and the Pacific, Bangkok 2, Thailand.

Library of Congress Cataloging-in-Publication Data

Retherford, Robert D.
    Comparison of fertility trends estimated alternatively
from birth histories and own children.

    (Papers of the East-West Population Institute ;
no. 94)
    Bibliography: p.
    1. Fertility, Human. 2. Demography—Methodology.
I. Alam, Iqbal. II. Title. III. Series.
HB901.R48   1985   304.6'32'072   85-13166
ISBN 0-86638-068-X

CONTENTS

FIGURES AND APPENDIX TABLE

Figures

Appendix Table

PREFACE

A preliminary version of this paper was presented at the World Fertility Survey Symposium, 24–27 April 1984, in London.

We are grateful to John Cleland, Thomas Pullum, and Chris Scott for helpful comments, and to Robin Loomis, Wayne Shima, Victoria Ho, and Judith Tom for research and computer programming assistance. Support for this research was provided by the United States Agency for International Development and the International Statistical Institute.

The views expressed herein are those of the authors and do not necessarily reflect the views of the United Nations.

ABSTRACT   Fertility trends estimated alternatively from birth histories and own children are compared for eight developing countries in which the World Fertility Survey was conducted. Principal hypotheses are that fertility trends estimated by the two approaches suffer from similar errors in the reporting of women's and children's ages, and that these errors are more severe in estimates derived from own children than in estimates derived from birth histories. The hypotheses are confirmed in four of the eight countries. Potter's hypothesis about misplacement of events toward the survey date, which assumes bunching of births five to ten years before the survey and accurate reporting of births during the first five years or so immediately preceding the survey, resulting in a spurious estimated fertility decline, does not receive much support from these data. Some of the estimated fertility declines do indeed seem spurious, but Potter's explanation of them seems inconsistent with the data. In some countries, patterns of age misreporting involving upward rounding of children's ages provide an equally plausible explanation that is more consistent with the data.

The birth history method and the own-children method are two major methods of estimating fertility trends from survey or census data. The birth history method has been used, for example, in the World Fertility Survey (WFS). The own-children method (Cho, 1973) has been applied mainly to censuses or large household surveys. This paper compares fertility trends estimated alternatively by these two methods.

It is well known that both birth history analysis and own-children analysis frequently provide distorted estimates of fertility trends. The reasons underlying such distortions are, however, imperfectly understood. In a widely cited article on estimating fertility trends from birth histories, Potter (1977) emphasized the role of event misplacement, which can lead to overestimating a decline in age-specific birth rates. He hypothesized that recent events are recorded fairly accurately, but more distant events are misplaced toward the date of interview. The consequence is an artificial bunching of events five to ten years before the survey that results in an estimated fertility decline during the ten years or so previous to the survey that is spuriously large. Event misplacement tends to be associated with misreporting of children's ages. For example, an erroneous response that a child's age is, say, 11 years may be associated in a very direct way with a parallel erroneous response that the child's date of birth was 11 years previous to the survey.

Event misplacement and associated misreporting of children's ages
are only part of the story. Analysis of data on own children suggests
that misreporting of adults' ages can also lead to major distortions in
fertility trends. For example, Retherford and Mirza (1982) have
shown that in Pakistan a pattern of age exaggeration that increases
with age for both children and adults could explain a pattern of
estimated fertility change whereby fertility declined substantially at
the older reproductive ages and increased substantially at most
younger ages during a period when other evidence suggests that very
little fertility change of any kind actually occurred. In contrast to
Potter's model, which assumes accurate fertility estimates for the first
five years or so immediately preceding the survey, age exaggeration of
children implies fertility underestimates during this same period. This
point of difference is elaborated later in this paper.

The principal hypothesis examined in this paper is that fertility
trends estimated alternatively from birth histories and own children
suffer from similar errors in the reporting of women's and children's
ages and therefore should show a similar pattern of distortions from
this source. It is hypothesized additionally that the distortions are less
pronounced in estimates of fertility trends derived from birth histories
than in those derived from own children. One expects this because the
interviewer has more opportunity to notice and correct internal inconsistencies (e.g., implausibly short birth intervals) when collecting birth
histories than when collecting own-children data. Moreover, questions
on ages of children are usually more extensive and probing in the birth
histories than in the household surveys. Furthermore, reporting by
surrogates is absent in birth histories, where mothers invariably report
for themselves and their children, but frequent in the household surveys, where the household head often responds for the entire household. A number of different methods of collecting birth histories were
employed in WFS surveys (Jemai and Singh, 1984), a fact that affects
the interpretation of findings presented later in this paper.

These hypotheses about similar sources of distortions in fertility
estimates derived from birth histories and own children are tested on
WFS data from eight developing countries: Dominican Republic,
Indonesia, Kenya, Korea, Nepal, Pakistan, Sri Lanka, and Syria. Each
of these country surveys covered a sample of either ever-married
women or, in the cases of Dominican Republic and Kenya, both ever-
married and single women, from whom birth histories were collected.

This sample, called the individual sample, was embedded in a larger sample of complete households, called the household sample. In this study, the fertility trend is estimated alternatively from birth histories from the individual sample and from own-children data from the household sample. The two estimated trends are then compared for each of the eight countries.

METHODOLOGY

In the birth history approach, age-specific totals of births to ever-married women are reconstructed from the birth histories for each year previous to the survey. Person-years of exposure to risk for ever-married women are similarly reconstructed. Except for Dominican Republic and Kenya, where the individual sample included both ever-married and single women, person-years at risk for all women, regardless of marital status, are estimated by dividing appropriate age-specific categories of person-years at risk for ever-married women by appropriate age-specific proportions ever-married at the time of the survey. These proportions ever-married are usually determined from the WFS household samples; thus the birth history analysis is usually not based entirely on the individual sample. In these computations, base calculations are done in century months, which are then aggregated to years or group of years as desired. The birth history approach ordinarily assumes that all births previous to the survey occurred to women who were ever-married at the time of the survey and that none occurred to women still single (never-married). It also assumes that women who died during the estimation period previous to the survey had, while they were alive, age-specific birth rates identical to those of women who survived. More detailed discussions of birth history analysis are found in numerous WFS publications (see, for example, Goldman, Coale, and Weinstein, 1979).

In this study, the WFS computer program package, FERTRATE, was used to generate fertility estimates from birth histories. The time periods for which estimates were calculated were counted backward in 12-month intervals starting from the time of the survey rather than from January 1 of the year of the survey, so that the estimates are comparable to those generated by the own-children method. The 12-month intervals are labeled by the calendar year that encompasses most of the interval; for example, the period June 1978–May 1979 would be labeled 1978, since more than half of the period falls in 1978.

The second approach to estimation utilizes the own-children method, which is a reverse-survival technique for estimating age-specific birth rates for years previous to a census or, in this instance, a household survey. Enumerated children are first matched to mothers within households, ordinarily on the basis of answers to questions on age, sex, marital status, number of children still living, and relation to head of household. WFS household surveys, however, contain a special code directly linking children to their mothers, so that matching can be accomplished quite simply. These matched (i.e., own) children, classified by own age and mother's age, are reverse-survived to estimate numbers of births by age of mother in previous years. Reverse-survival is also used to estimate numbers of women by age in previous years. After adjustments are made for unmatched (non-own) children, age-specific birth rates are calculated by dividing the number of births by the number of women. Estimates are computed for each previous year or groups of years back to 15 years before the survey. Estimates are not computed further back than 15 years because births must then be based on children aged 15 or older at enumeration, a large proportion of whom do not reside in the same household as their mother and hence cannot be matched. Data for women up to age 65 at enumeration are utilized, in order that birth rates for the full reproductive age range 15–49 can be calculated for every year up to the 15th year before the survey. All calculations are done initially by single years of age and time. Estimates for groups of ages or groups of calendar years are obtained by appropriately aggregating numerators and denominators of single-year rates and then dividing the aggregated numerator by the aggregated denominator.

Unmatched (non-own) children are allocated to mothers by multiplying each age-specific category of matched (own) children, specified by mother's age, by the corresponding age-specific ratio of all children to own children. Thus own children of a given age are adjusted upward by the same factor regardless of mother's age, thereby introducing some error in the fertility estimates since the proportionate distribution of non-own children by age of mother generally differs somewhat from the proportionate distribution of own children by age of mother. Since older women are usually in more stable household situations than younger women, the nature of this error is usually to reallocate a certain proportion of non-own children of a given age from younger mothers to older mothers. This error, if it occurs, usually has little effect on the total fertility rate, but it produces an age pattern of fertility that is too low at the younger ages and too high at the older ages. The adjustment factors for non-own children are usually low enough that this bias is slight. Further details of the own-children method may be found in Cho (1973) and Retherford and Cho (1978).

As mentioned, the own-children method requires life tables, from which reverse-survival ratios are computed. For Dominican Republic, Korea, and Syria, constant mortality over time was assumed, and life tables were calculated by matching child mortality estimates obtained by applying Brass's (1975) method to child survivorship data (numbers of children ever born and still living by age of mother) from the WFS survey itself, to the appropriate Coale-Demeny Model West life table (Coale and Demeny, 1966). For Indonesia, changing mortality was assumed. Estimates of life expectancy for 1960 and 1978 were obtained from the United Nations 1976 and 1981 Demographic Yearbooks and were matched to Coale-Demeny Model West life tables. These life tables were interpolated to single years of age and time by procedures described in Retherford (1978) and Retherford and Cho (1978). A similar procedure was used for Kenya, except that the starting estimates for life expectancy were for 1969 and 1978. For Nepal, we began with life expectancy estimates of 37.5 for 1960 and 42.5 for 1975 and then used the same procedure followed for Indonesia and Kenya. For Pakistan, constant mortality was assumed, and the life table used was that derived from the Population Growth Estimation (PGE) Survey of 1962–65 (Afzal, 1974:22). For Sri Lanka, constant mortality was assumed, and published life tables for 1970–72 were used (Sri Lanka Department of Census and Statistics, 1978).

The own-children estimates are rather insensitive to errors in the mortality estimates, because such errors cause only very small changes in reverse-survival ratios, which under modern mortality conditions are always rather close to one, even in developing countries (Retherford, Chamratrithirong, and Wanglee, 1980). For the countries examined here, errors in the fertility estimates due to mortality estimation errors are much smaller than the errors stemming from age misreporting that are the focus of this report. Moreover, the method of mortality estimation guarantees an absence of mortality fluctuations over time during the estimation period. Thus there is no danger whatever that year-to-year distortions in the estimated fertility trends examined here could be due to mortality estimation errors.

No adjustments for incorrect enumeration (age-selective sampling bias or age misreporting) are made, either in the birth history analysis or in the own-children analysis, since these are the phenomena we wish to observe.

As mentioned, the own-children data include information on women up to 65 years of age. In the birth histories, however, only women below age 50 were queried. This means that, for the 15-year estimation period previous to the survey (the focus of this report), annual estimates of complete age-specific fertility schedules covering the entire reproductive age range 15–49 can be computed from the own-children data but not from the birth history data, which suffer from truncation as soon as one considers time periods previous to the survey. For example, if one wishes to compute age-specific birth rates for the fifth year previous to the survey from the birth histories, one is restricted to women aged 15–44 at that time instead of the full range 15–49. For the full 15-year estimation period, the range is restricted to ages 15–34. This means that the most desirable fertility measure, the total fertility rate, cannot be used in comparing fertility trends estimated by the two methods. Instead, we use the cumulative fertility rate at exact age 35, CFR(35), which is calculated as five times the sum of age-specific birth rates for age groups 15–19 through 30–34. Note the similarity to the total fertility rate, which is calculated in the same way but with a higher age cutoff. It will also be of interest to examine trends in age-specific birth rates.

THE WFS DATA

For this study, the WFS samples examined here may be categorized into three groups:

Group 1

In the first group, which is the largest, the household and individual samples are the same in that every woman in the individual sample belongs to a household in the household sample, and every eligible woman in every household of the household sample belongs to the individual sample (except for those few eligible women who were nonrespondents in the individual survey). Additionally, in this group's surveys, field operations were carried out at approximately the same time and by the same field staff. Nepal, Pakistan, and Sri Lanka are in this group.

Given the almost simultaneous timing of the individual and household interviews for these countries, one might expect a close correspondence between the two samples in reported ages and birth dates. Preliminary tabulations indicated, however, that this was not always the case. Our explanation for this lack of agreement hypothesizes the following sequence of events: Ages of all household members were first collected in the household interview. From the household schedule, ever-married women were identified. These women were subsequently questioned and birth histories collected in individual interviews. In the process of collecting birth histories, there was intensive questioning about birth intervals and dating of events, resulting in some cases, by implication, in improved estimates of the respondent's or her children's ages. But these improved estimates are reflected in the household survey results only to the extent that someone, either in the field or in the office, took the trouble to go back to the household schedules and render the reports of women's and children's ages consistent with birth dates recorded in the birth histories. Apparently this was done much more completely in some countries than in others, and in some cases it may not have been done at all (Jemai and Singh, 1984).

We have no way of knowing the extent of consistency checking and resolving of discrepancies that actually occurred, and this uncertainty results in an unknown degree of contamination that obscures the meaning of the comparisons to be made. The results for Pakistan and Nepal, however, suggest that little consistency checking was done, so that the comparisons seem unambiguous. In Sri Lanka, the third country in this group, age reporting is comparatively good, and there seems to be little consequent distortion in the trend estimates derived by either method.

The numbers of ever-married women in the individual sample and persons in the household sample are 5,940 and 31,971 for Nepal, 4,952 and 32,008 for Pakistan, and 6,810 and 47,914 for Sri Lanka.

Group 2

In this category the individual sample is a subsample of the household sample, with the latter generally covering three or four times as many households as the former. The two surveys were carried out at approximately the same time and by the same field staff so that contamination is not excluded, but it is clearly less serious than in the countries in Group 1 because it can only affect the minority of mothers who were selected for the individual survey. In this study, three countries fall in Group 2: Dominican Republic, Korea, and Syria. In the Dominican Republic, the women in the individual sample were sampled directly from a list of all the eligible women in the household sample (i.e., there was no process of subsampling households). In Korea and Syria, the individual sample consists of all eligible women in a subsample of the households of the household sample.

The numbers of ever-married women in the individual sample and persons in the household sample are 3,115 and 59,493 for Dominican Republic, 5,430 and 104,892 for Korea, and 4,487 and 97,310 for Syria.

Group 3

In this group, the individual and household schedules (the household schedule was very short) were administered in the same interview, so that this case represents the most extreme form of contamination of any of the three groups. Indonesia and Kenya fall in this category. In the case of Indonesia, however, this difficulty can largely be circumvented, because the WFS household survey, known as SUPAS III, was embedded in a much larger survey known as SUPAS II. Thus fertility trends can be estimated by the own-children method from SUPAS II as well as SUPAS III, both of which will be examined in this paper. Because of the large sample size of SUPAS II, the own-children fertility estimates derived from it are relatively free of contamination. No such remedy for contamination is available to us for Kenya, and the results for Kenya are therefore less instructive than those for the other countries.

The numbers of ever-married women in the individual sample and persons in the household sample are 9,155 and 50,994 for Indonesia and 8,100 and 46,101 for Kenya. The SUPAS II sample, of which the WFS household sample, SUPAS III, is a subsample, contains 281,168 persons.

FINDINGS

Findings are presented in the order of the three groups discussed previously. Trends in age-specific birth rates and cumulative fertility rates to age 35, CFR(35), estimated alternatively from birth histories and own children, are given in Appendix Table 1. Figure 1 summarizes this table by graphing trends in CFR(35), and Figure 2 by graphing trends in age-specific birth rates. In each case, trends are estimated alternatively from birth histories and own children.

Results for Nepal are presented in Panel A of Figures 1 and 2. The CFR estimates derived by the own-children method in Panel A of Figure 1 show a pattern that has been found to be fairly typical for countries of continental South Asia, namely large oscillations during the period 10–14 years before the survey and a substantial fertility decline during the 8 years or so immediately preceding the survey. Usually the estimates show a fertility upturn in the year just preceding the survey, and this is also evident for Nepal.

The large oscillations during the period 10–14 years before the survey reflect severe heaping on children's ages 10 and 12, corresponding to births in the 11th and 13th years before the survey. The comparatively low fertility during the first five years or so immediately preceding the survey may be due mainly to age exaggeration from rounding of children's ages to the next higher age. For example, at age 0 (corresponding to the first year before the survey), it is possible that many children of 11 months and perhaps younger ages as well are rounded to 1 year of age, resulting in a deficit of children at age 0 and a corresponding underestimate of cumulative fertility for the first year before the survey. At age 1 (corresponding to the second year before the survey), substantial rounding to two years may occur not only at 23 months of age but also at 22 and 21 months and perhaps even younger ages as well. Thus the tendency to round upward from age 1 to age 2 may be greater than the tendency to round upward from age 0 to age 1, resulting in an overall deficit at age 1. Upward rounding that is substantially more pronounced for 1-year-olds than for 0-year-olds may explain the frequent and often spurious finding that cumulative fertility is lower in the second year before the survey than in the first year. At ages 2, 3, . . . , 8, it is plausible that the rate at which upward rounding increases with age diminishes with age, so that estimated fertility increases as one moves backward in time. At ages beyond 8 (corresponding to nine or more years before the survey), heaping on ages 8, 10, and 12 predominates, resulting in sharp peaks in the CFR trend during the 9th, 11th, and 13th years before the survey.

The parallel CFR trend based on birth histories for Nepal in Panel A of Figure 1 bears only a slight resemblance to that based on own

10

FIGURE 1. Trends in cumulative fertility rates, CFR(35), estimated alternatively from birth histories and own children

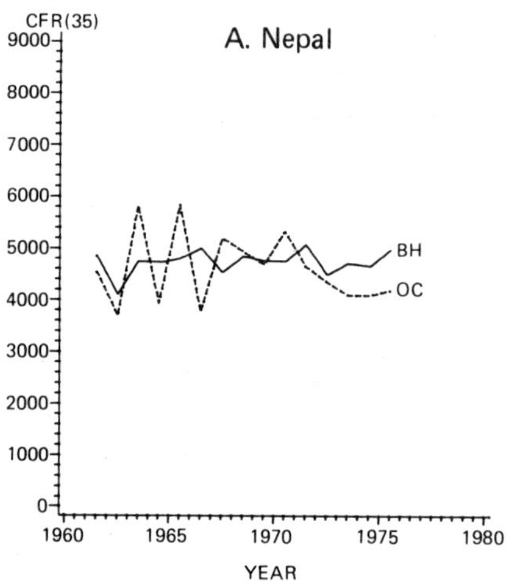

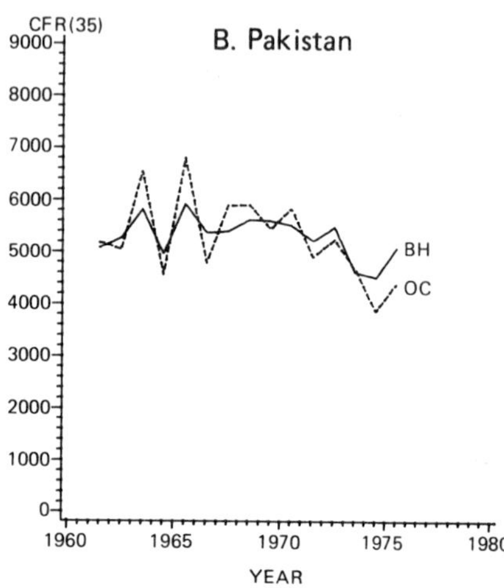

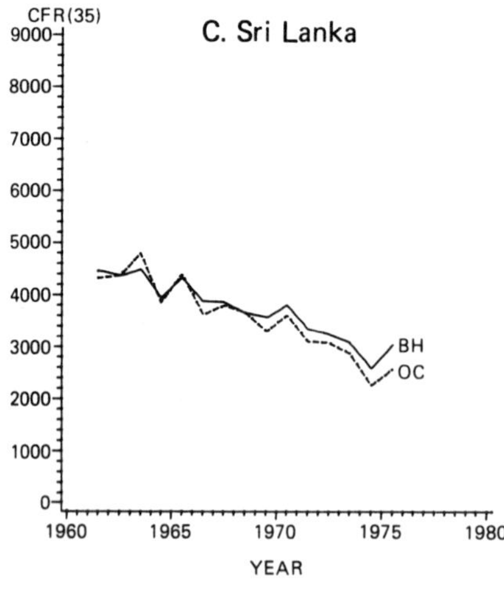

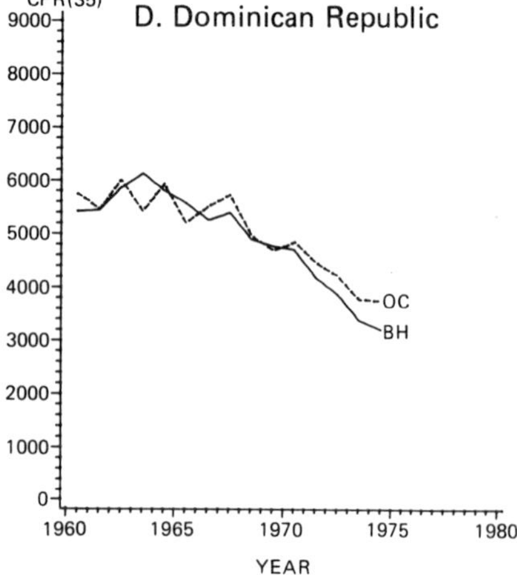

FIGURE 1. *(continued)*

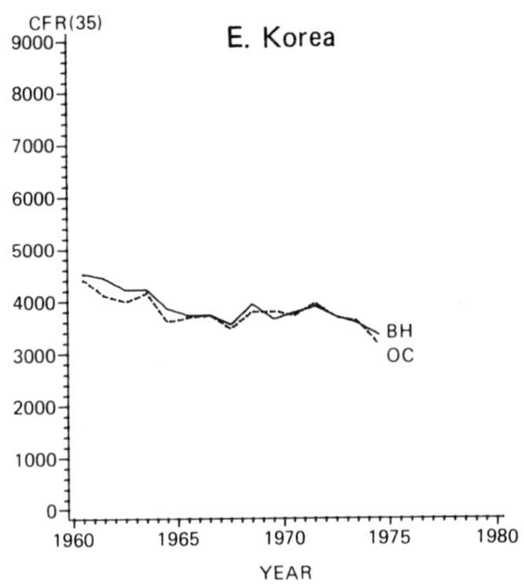

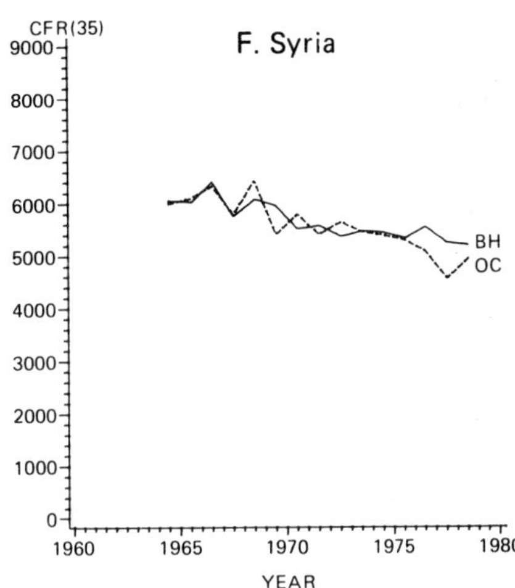

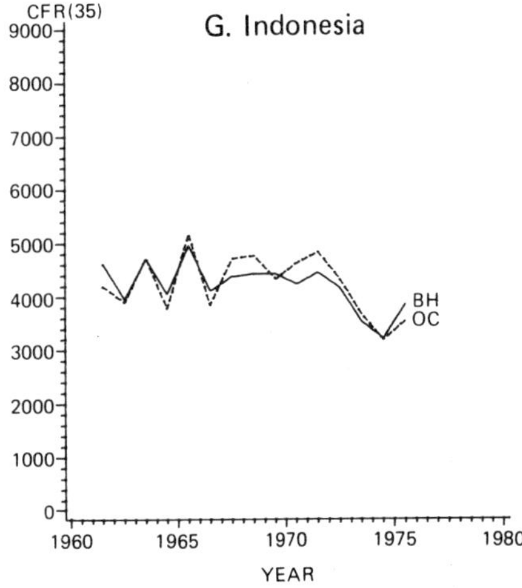

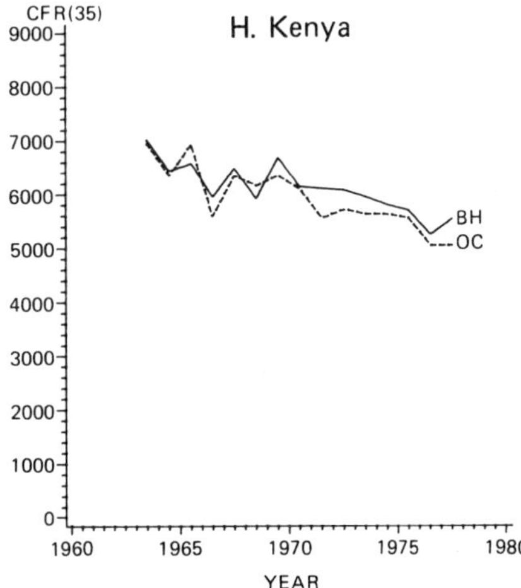

FIGURE 2. Trends in age-specific birth rates estimated alternatively from birth histories and own children

A. Nepal

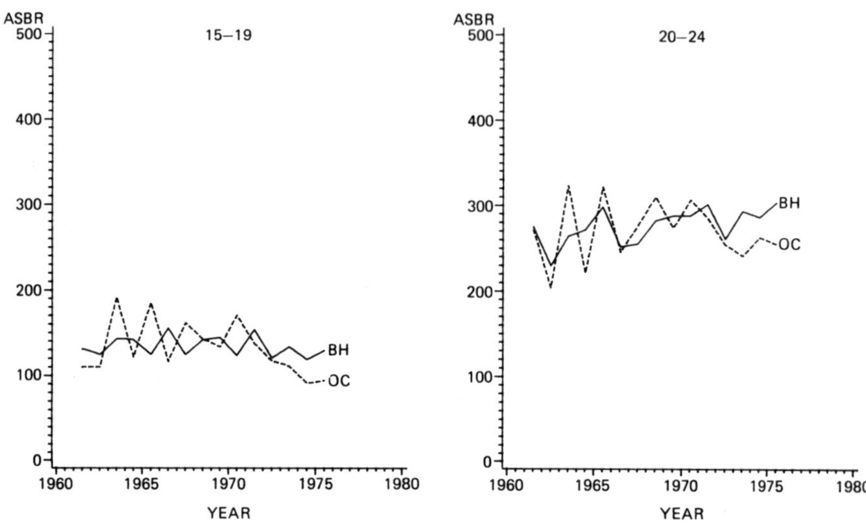

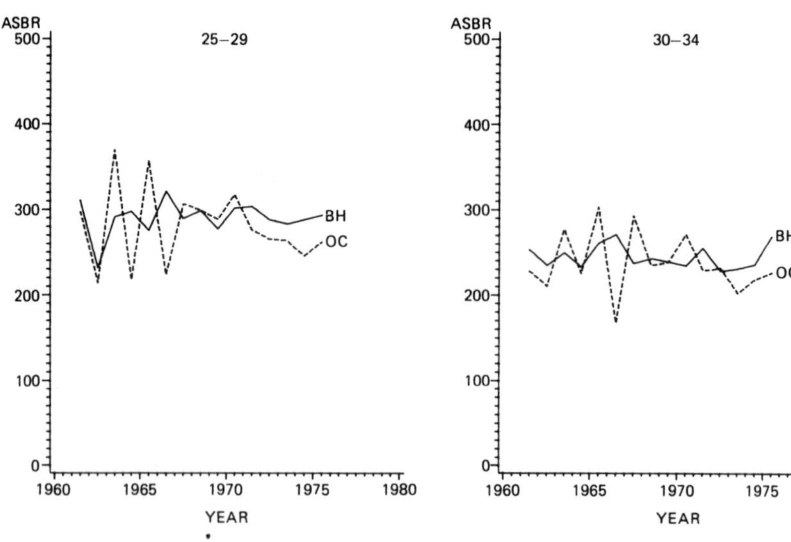

FIGURE 2.   *(continued)*

B. Pakistan

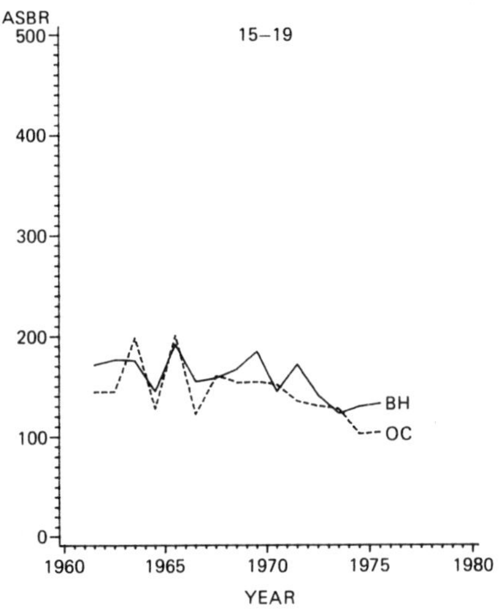

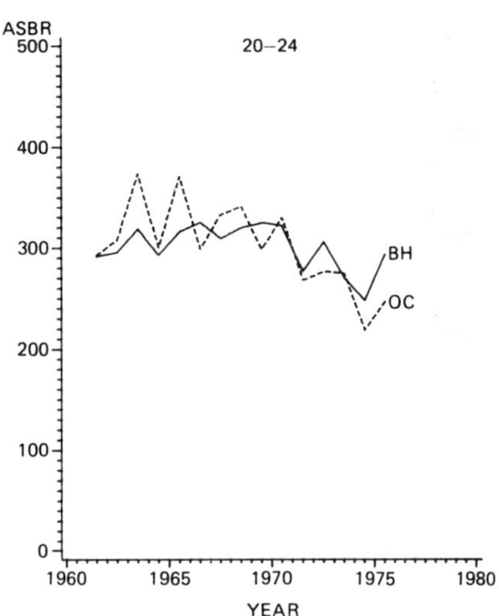

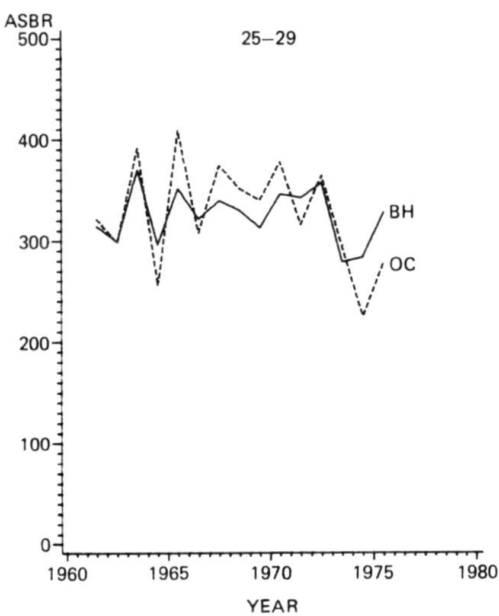

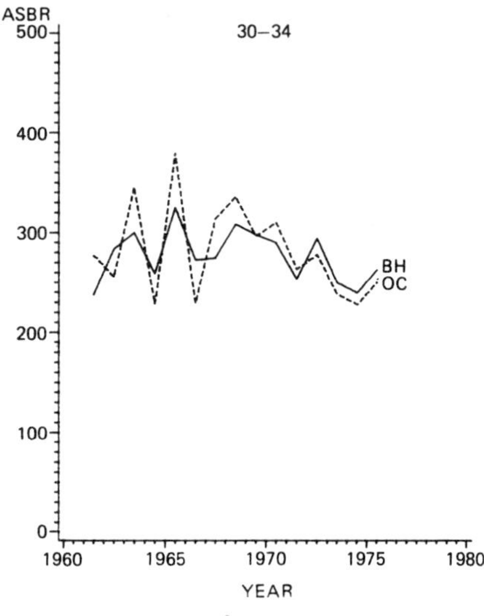

14

FIGURE 2. *(continued)*

C. Sri Lanka

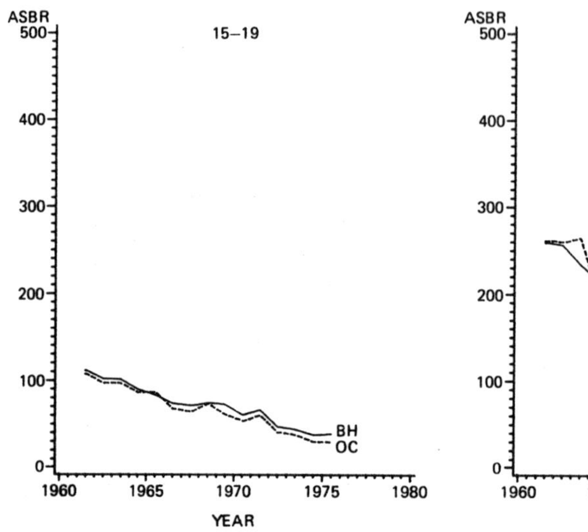

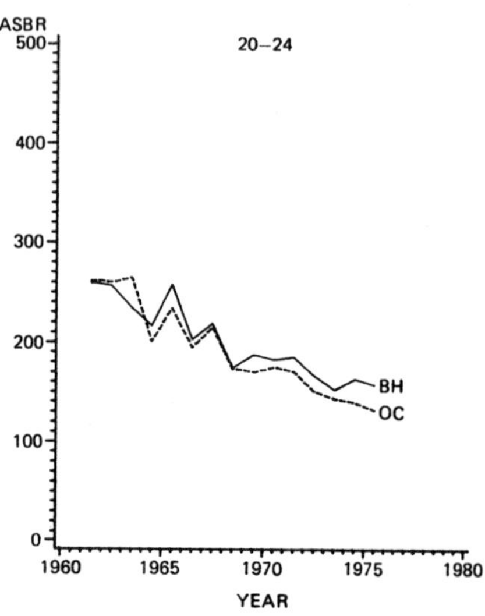

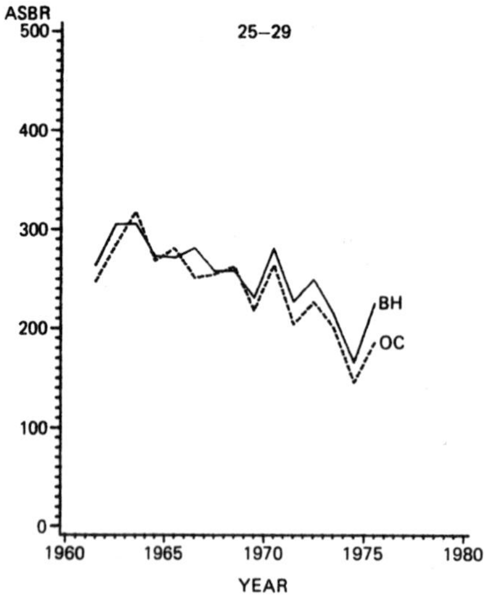

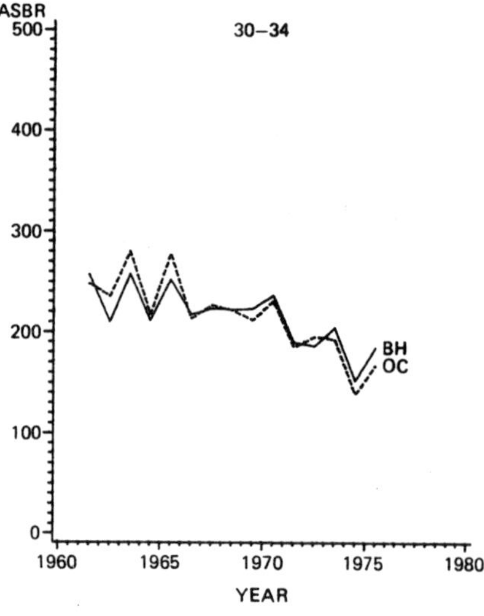

FIGURE 2. *(continued)*

D. Dominican Republic

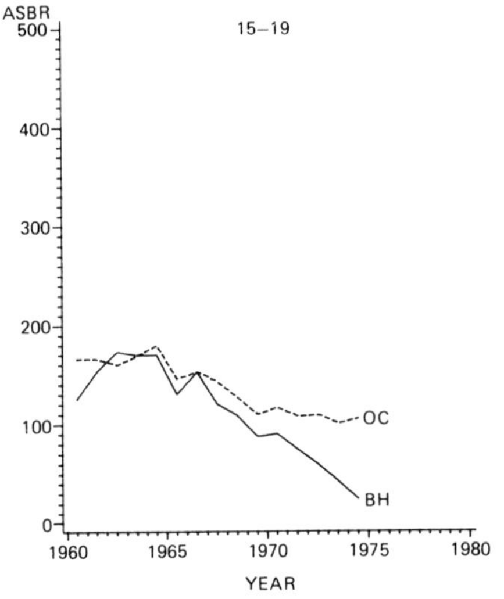

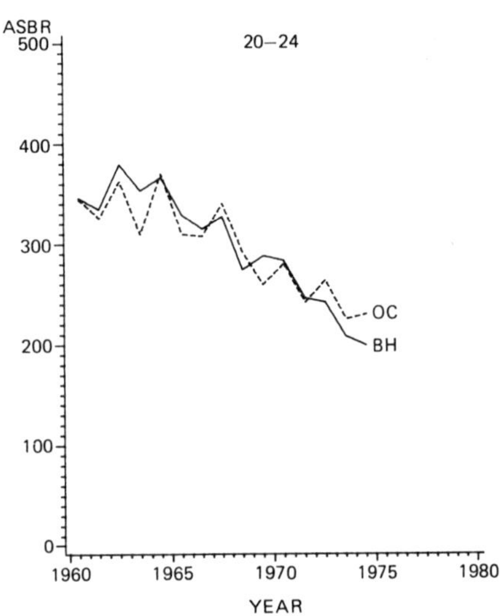

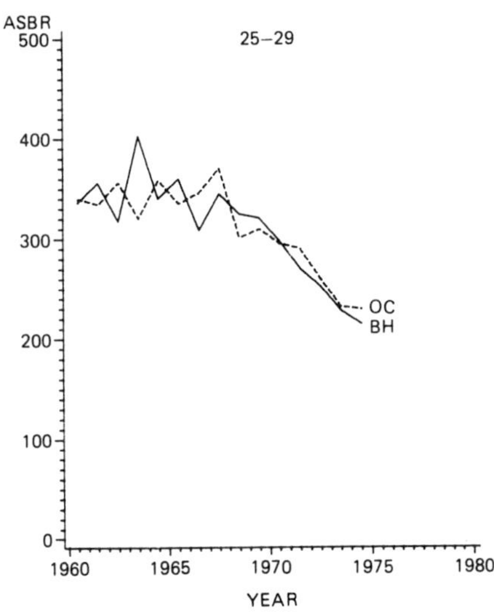

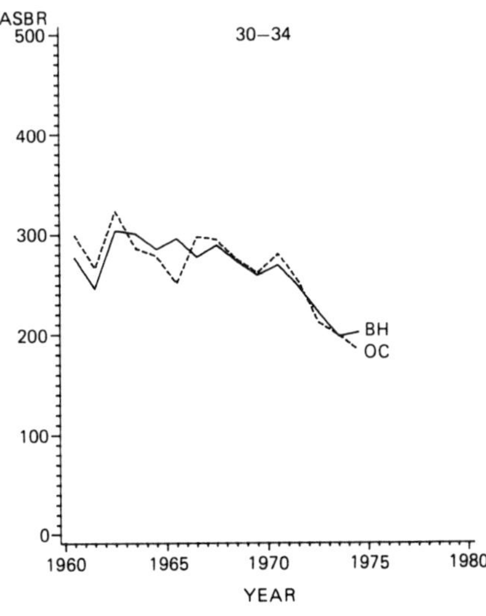

16

FIGURE 2. *(continued)*

E. Korea

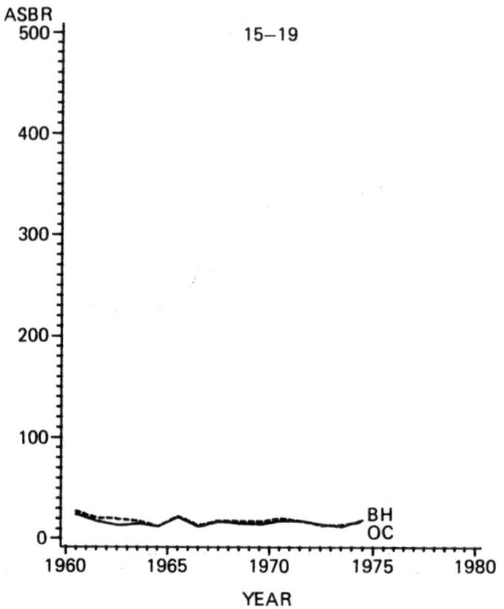

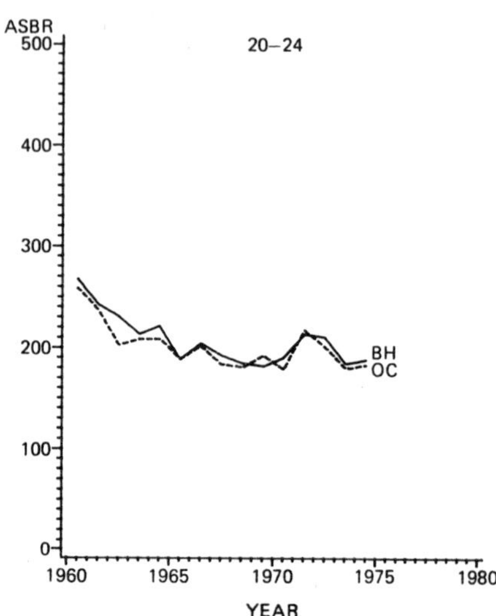

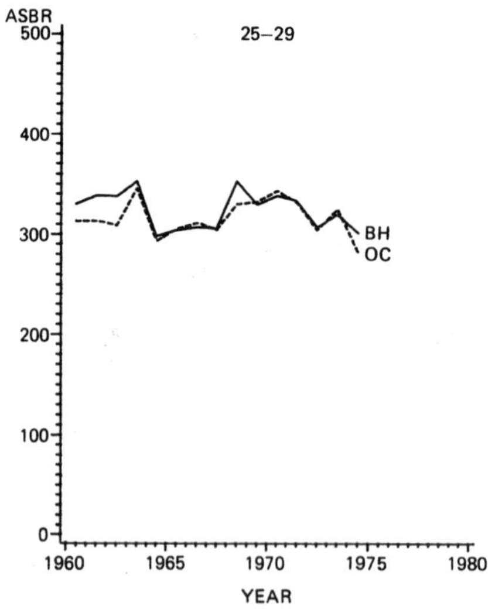

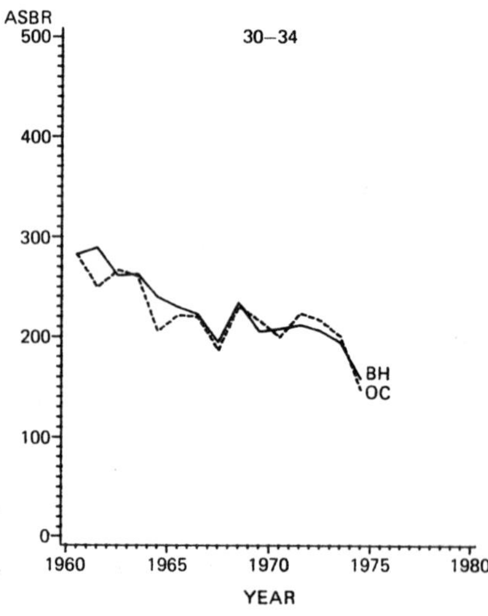

FIGURE 2. *(continued)*

F. Syria

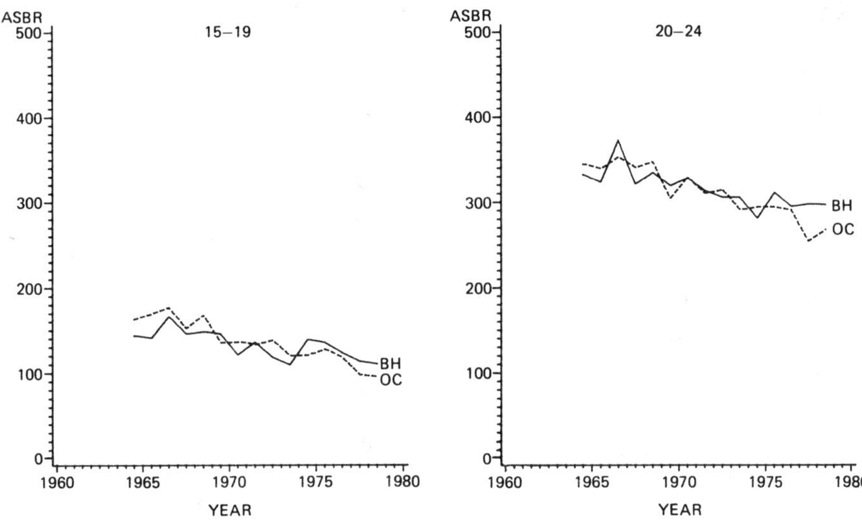

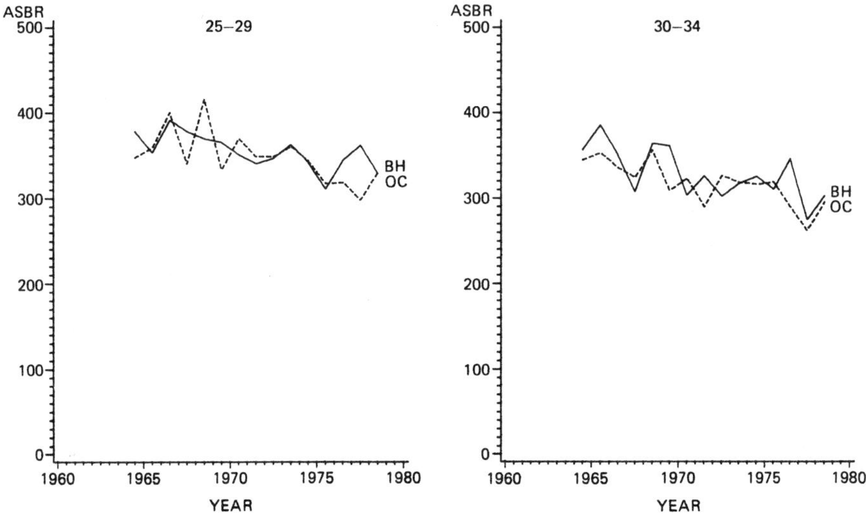

FIGURE 2. *(continued)*

G. Indonesia

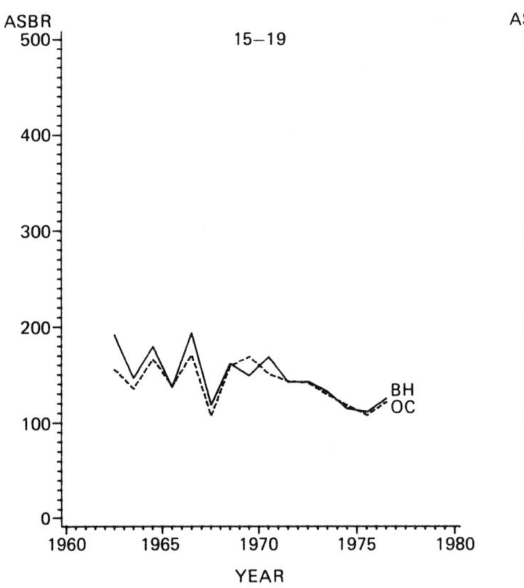

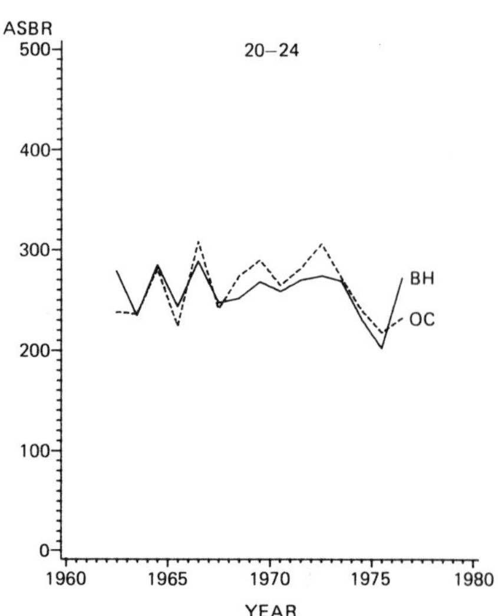

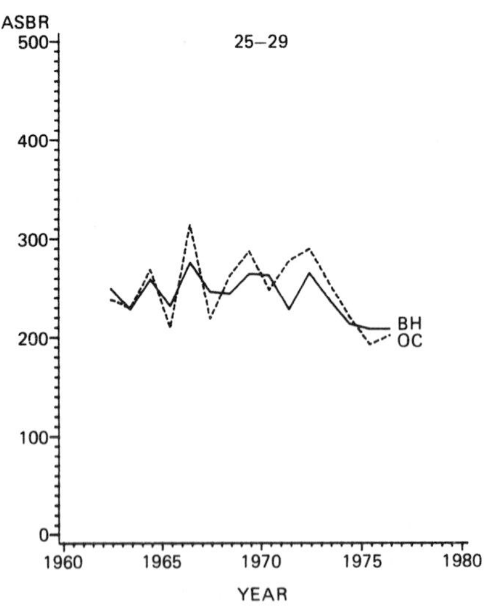

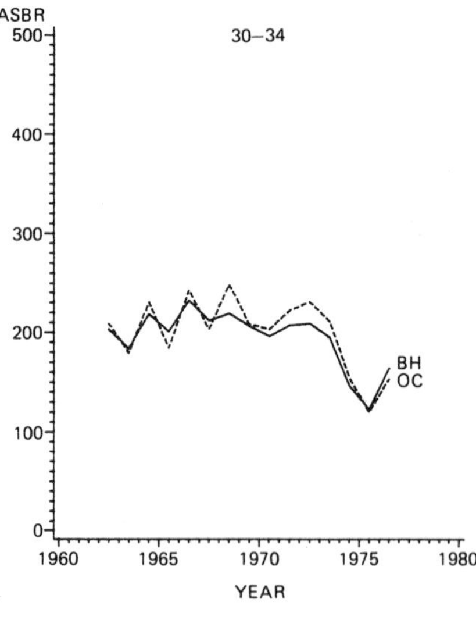

FIGURE 2. *(continued)*

H. Kenya

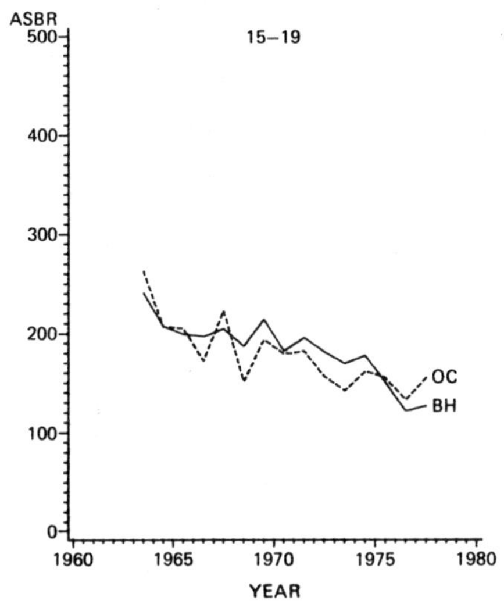

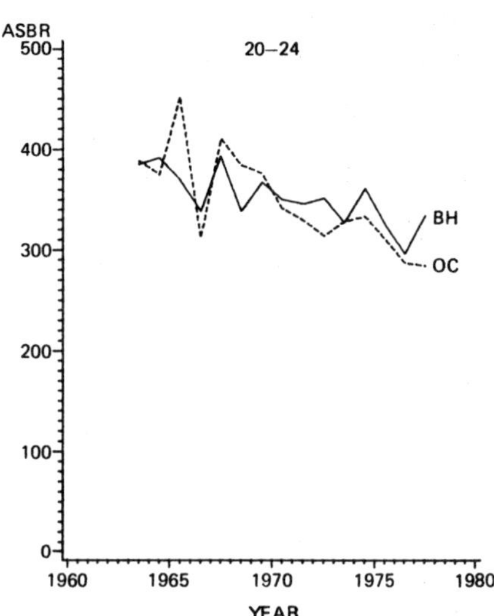

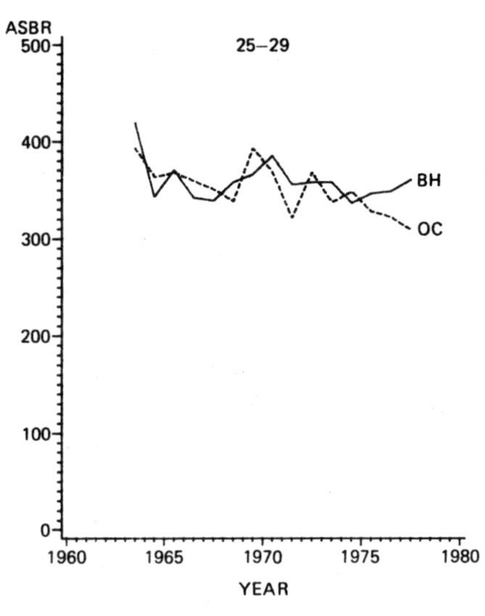

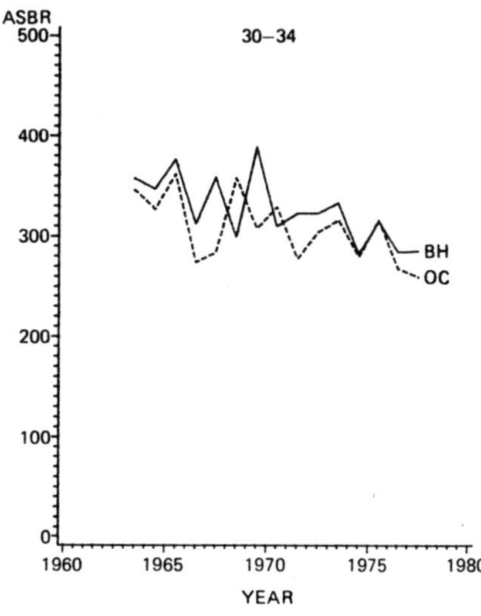

children. On the whole, the estimates based on birth histories show little change over time, indicating an absence of fertility decline, and the comparatively minor year-to-year fluctuations do not parallel very closely those derived from own children. The results seem either to contradict our hypothesis that fertility trends based alternatively on birth histories and own children reflect the same age reporting errors, or to suggest that the survey takers made exceptional efforts, through probing, to achieve a degree of consistency in the reporting of the timing of birth events in the birth histories that left few traces of age misreporting.

The impressively smooth results from birth histories may have something to do with the Takeshita method of collecting birth histories. This method, which was used in Nepal but not in most other WFS countries, makes special efforts to obtain accurate age data (Jemai and Singh, 1984). The smooth results from the birth histories may also be related to extensive imputation of dates of events collected in the birth histories (Chidambaram and Sathar, forthcoming). But imputation cannot be the main reason for the smooth trend from the Nepalese birth histories, because, as we shall see, this trend is much less smooth in Pakistan, where imputation was just as extensive as in Nepal. If age misreporting is the principal cause of whatever year-to-year distortions remain in the fertility trend estimates for Nepal, then it is apparent that little or no effort was made to render birth dates in the individual sample and ages in the household sample consistent with each other.

Panel A of Figure 2 for Nepal shows similar graphs for age-specific birth rates. The pattern is rather similar to that for the CFR in Figure 1, except that the graphs are considerably more jagged for older women than for younger women. We interpret this to mean that older women provide less accurate reports of ages and birth dates for themselves and their children than do younger women.

Panel B in Figure 1 and 2 shows results for Pakistan. The pattern of own-children estimates is quite similar to that for Nepal, with pronounced fertility fluctuations early in the estimation period, substantial fertility decline subsequently, and a small upturn in the year immediately preceding the survey; but age misreporting seems more severe, as indicated by more jagged patterns. Again major peaks in the fertility trend occur in the 11th and 13th years previous to the survey, corresponding to heaping on ages 10 and 12. Consonant with our initial hypothesis, the fertility trends estimated by the own-children method are considerably more jagged than those estimated from birth histories, and they show a similar pattern of year-to-year fluctuations. Peaks and troughs in the estimated trends derived by the two methods coincide rather closely. Regarding age-specific birth rates, this similarity is especially striking for the older age groups 25–29 and 30–34. Thus the Pakistan data tend to support our hypothesis that fertility trends estimated alternatively from birth histories and own children suffer from similar biases due to similar age reporting errors in both data sets.

In Pakistan as in Nepal, independent evidence from the WFS on contraceptive use rates, which are below 5 percent, suggests that very little real fertility decline occurred over the estimation periods considered here. Whatever real fertility decline did occur in Pakistan was almost certainly confined largely to the 15–19 age group, owing to a slow but steady rise in mean age at marriage over the past two decades. Yet Panel B of Figure 2 shows estimated fertility declines during the five years or so immediately preceding the survey that are as great or greater at the older reproductive ages as at 15–19. This suggests that the estimated fertility declines are largely spurious.

Results for the third country in Group 1, Sri Lanka, are shown in Panel C of Figures 1 and 2. The trends estimated alternatively from birth histories and own children show annual fluctuations that tend to rise and fall together, and this pattern again supports our hypothesis that the two trends are similarly biased by age reporting errors. There tend to be peaks in the 6th, 9th, 11th, and 13th years before the survey, corresponding to heaping on ages 5, 8, 10, and 12. The heaping is comparatively minor, however, in keeping with the comparatively accurate age reporting that is known to characterize Sri Lanka (Ratnayake, Retherford, and Sivasubramaniam, 1984). Heaping is considerably worse for older than for younger women, and this probably reflects much better age reporting by younger women. The sharp gradient in the quality of age reporting between older and younger women may in turn be related to the rapid improvement in public education in Sri Lanka over the previous two decades, particularly for women.

In Sri Lanka as well as in Nepal and Pakistan, there tends to be a small fertility upturn in the year immediately preceding the survey. Overall, the recurring pattern of fertility peaks corresponding to children's ages 0, 8, 10, and 12 strongly suggests that the observed peaks and troughs in the fertility trends are primarily due to age misreporting and do not reflect real annual fluctuations in fertility. (Note, however, that sampling errors for single-year rates are large; see Little, 1982.)

We now come to the Group 2 countries, for which, it will be recalled, the individual sample is embedded in a considerably larger household sample. Results for Dominican Republic are shown in Panel D of Figures 1 and 2. Figure 1 shows that trends estimated alternatively from birth histories and own children coincide reasonably closely, except for the five years immediately preceding the survey, where fertility declines more steeply for the birth history estimates than for the own-children estimates. In the estimates derived by the own-children method, there appears to be some heaping on ages 4, 7, 10, and 12, corresponding to local peaks in the fertility trend in the 5th, 8th, 11th, and 13th years before the survey. (Nepal, Pakistan, and Sri Lanka, it will be recalled, also showed heaping on ages 10 and 12.) The trend estimated from birth histories also shows local peaks in the 5th and 8th years before the survey, but not in the 11th and 13th years; instead, it peaks in the 12th year before the survey. Age reporting errors, described in a previous WFS study (Guzman, 1980), are implicated in these patterns, despite their inconsistencies.

Panel D of Figure 2 shows that the relatively steep fertility decline estimated from birth histories during the five years immediately preceding the survey is due mainly to discrepancies between the birth history and own-children trends at maternal ages 15–19, much less so to discrepancies at ages 20–24, and hardly at all to discrepancies at ages 25–29 and 30–34. Possibly age-specific proportions ever-married from the household sample were underestimated at the younger reproductive ages, resulting in an excessive deflation of birth rates for ever-married women at these ages when these latter rates were effectively multiplied through by age-specific proportions ever-married to estimate birth rates for women of all marital statuses combined. Such an error would result in fertility underestimates derived from the birth histories. Given well-known difficulties in assessing the extent of consensual unions (which are especially prevalent at the younger reproductive ages) as opposed to formal unions in many Caribbean countries, this seems a plausible source of error.

The relatively smooth estimated fertility decline since 1965 in the

Dominican Republic suggests that age misreporting problems are not severe and that the downward trend in fertility is real. This impression is reinforced by information on contraceptive use rates, which the WFS found to be substantial: 97 percent of eligible women knew of at least one modern contraceptive method, and 26 percent were using one (Hobcraft and Rodriguez, 1982).

It is noteworthy that fertility in Dominican Republic declines fastest at the peak reproductive ages, 20–24 and 25–29, indicating that birth control for both spacing and limiting started at about the same time. This pattern, while not unprecedented, is not the most common pattern observed in developing countries, where fertility more usually declines first at 15–19, due to rising age at marriage (more common in Asia than in Latin America), and at ages above 30, due to limiting behavior, and only somewhat later at 20–24 and 25–29 when birth control for spacing children starts to spread.

Results for Korea, the second country in Group 2, are shown in Panel E of Figures 1 and 2. In Figure 1, the CFR shows a decline in the 1960s, a temporary rise in the late 1960s and early 1970s, and resumption of decline in the 1970s. The temporary fertility resurgence in the late 1960s and early 1970s has also been observed in fertility trends estimated from other sources (see, for example, Retherford, Cho, and Kim, 1983) and seems to be real. The resurgence is most noticeable for age-specific birth rates at ages 20–24 and 25–29, as shown in Figure 2, which suggests that the resurgence was due to shifts in the timing of births due to unprecedented prosperity in the late 1960s and early 1970s, rather than to a temporary reversal of the downward trend of completed fertility. Age reporting is known to be very accurate in Korea, and there is no indication in Figures 1 and 2 that the small annual fluctuations in the two sets of fertility trends based alternatively on birth histories and own children reflect common patterns of age misreporting, which is largely absent.[1]

---

1. There appear to be errors in the current version of the Korea household tape. The proportions ever-married by single years of age computed from the tape do not agree with those published in the First Country Report. The proportions from the current tape are substantially too low at the younger reproductive ages and therefore yield fertility estimates from birth histories that are substantially too low. The proportions from the First Country Report, which agree closely with similar proportions computed from the 1975 Census, appear to be correct and were used instead for computing birth rates for all women (i.e., all marital statuses combined) from the birth histories. Another

Results for Syria, the third country in Group 2, are shown in Panel
F of Figures 1 and 2. The CFR trends estimated alternatively from
birth histories and own children in Figure 1 show quite good agreement during all but the most recent three years of the estimation
period, where the trend from own children drops below the trend
from birth histories. This pattern of coincidence and discrepancy
tends to be reflected also in the age-specific birth rate trends in
Figure 2, especially at the peak reproductive ages 20–24 and 25–29.
The peaks and troughs of the fertility trends estimated alternatively
from birth histories and own children do not coincide very con-
sistently.

As mentioned, the Group 3 countries, Indonesia and Kenya, have
the greatest degree of mutual contamination between birth histories
and own children, since both the individual and household schedules
were administered during the same interview. We examine Indonesia
first, in Panel G of Figures 1 and 2. As anticipated, the peaks and
troughs of the fertility trends estimated alternatively from birth histories and own children coincide rather well, and, as hypothesized,
the oscillations over time between peaks and troughs tend to be more
pronounced for the own-children estimates than for the birth history
estimates. The pattern of peaks and troughs resembles that for Nepal
and Pakistan, discussed earlier, namely peaks corresponding to children's ages 10 and 12 and an apparent fertility decline in the five
years or so immediately preceding the survey with a slight upturn in
the year just before the survey.

As mentioned earlier, an additional comparison is possible in the
case of Indonesia, because the WFS household sample, known as
SUPAS III, was embedded in a much larger household survey known
as SUPAS II. Figure 3 compares own-children estimates of trends in
the total fertility rate (TFR), covering the entire reproductive age
range 15–49, derived from SUPAS II and SUPAS III. The figure
shows that the pattern of peaks and troughs due to age misreporting
is quite similar in the two surveys, but it is considerably more

---

discrepancy is that the current household tape contains 1,232 more ever-
married women and 1,482 more persons than the household sample as reported in the First Country Report. We have not been able to pinpoint the
errors in the household tape, and it is possible that they also distort somewhat
the fertility estimates derived by the own-children method that are reported
here. Staff of the International Statistical Institute are currently investigating
this problem.

FIGURE 3. Trends in total fertility rates estimated by the own-children method: SUPAS II and SUPAS III, Indonesia

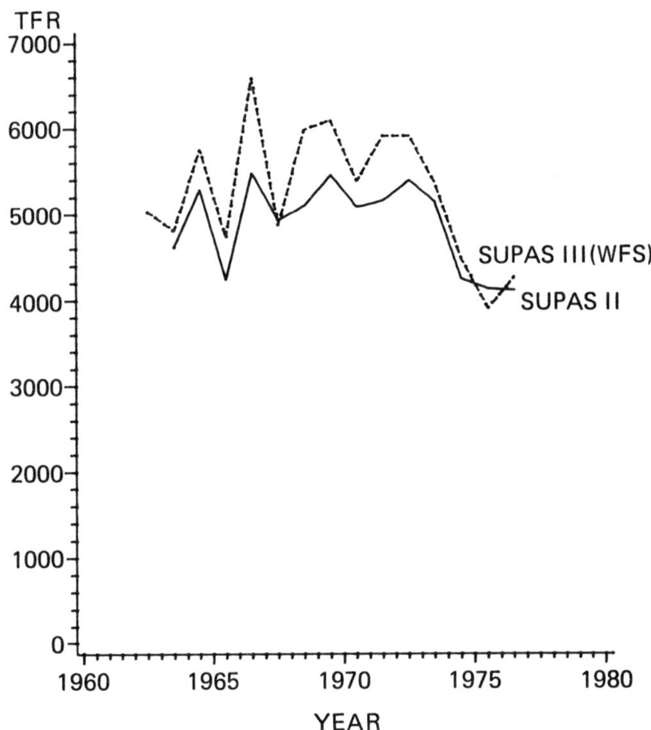

pronounced in SUPAS II than in the WFS SUPAS III. This pattern of discrepancies again tends to support our hypothesis that the collection of birth histories results in a good deal of internal consistency checking that ultimately provides better, or at least more consistent, estimates of women's and children's ages and the timing of birth events. The age-event chart used as an aid in collecting birth histories in Indonesia, as in Nepal, probably contributed to the quality of the age data obtained (Jemai and Singh, 1984; Supraptilah, 1982).

The last country in Group 3, and the last to be considered in this study, is Kenya, fertility trends for which are shown in Panel H of Figures 1 and 2. Again contamination between the individual and household samples is severe. As in the case of Indonesia, the CFR(35) trends estimated alternatively from birth histories and own children coincide rather well, although the trend derived from own children tends to be somewhat lower than the trend derived from birth histories in the first seven years or so immediately preceding the survey. Again there is some indication of heaping on ages 8, 10, and 12, corresponding to fertility peaks in the 9th, 11th, and 13th years before the survey; a subsequent decline in fertility; and a slight upturn in the year just preceding the survey. But this pattern is somewhat inconsistent when one examines the age-specific birth rate trends in Figure 2, and perhaps not too much significance should be attached to it. As in the other countries, year-to-year fluctuations tend to be larger in the own-children estimates than in the birth history estimates. Again this suggests that even though the household and individual schedules were administered in the same interview, birth dates and ages were not always rendered consistent in the two schedules. The data for Kenya tend also to support our original hypothesis that distortions in fertility trends estimated alternatively from birth histories and own children reflect similar age reporting errors. The quality of age data in the Kenyan WFS may have been enhanced by unusually detailed probes on age; however, age heaping in the WFS is not markedly different from age heaping in a previous survey that did not include such probes (Jemai and Singh, 1984; Henin, Korten, and Werner, 1982).

CONCLUSION

From the ages of surviving children matched to a woman in the own-children procedure, one can infer birth dates, yielding a partial birth history that omits births who later died or moved out of the household before being enumerated in the survey. In effect, the own-children adjustments for mortality and unmatched children compensate for these omissions. Thus the own-children method may be regarded as fertility estimation from incomplete maternity histories.

Given this similarity between the own-children method and the birth history method, the initial hypothesis of this paper was that fertility trends estimated alternatively from birth histories and own children tend to suffer from similar errors in age reporting that should be reflected in roughly coinciding peaks and troughs in the estimated year-to-year fertility trends. It was further hypothesized that the distortions due to age misreporting should be more pronounced in the trend derived from own children than in the trend derived from birth histories, since the latter offer more opportunity to detect and correct internal inconsistencies while interviewing respondents. These hypotheses are supported fairly strongly by the results for Pakistan, Sri Lanka, Indonesia, and Kenya, but only weakly or not at all by the results for Nepal, Dominican Republic, Korea, and Syria. In the case of Nepal, we speculate that an extraordinary effort was made to obtain birth histories with a smooth sequence of birth intervals, and that this effort left little trace of the typical South Asian pattern of age misreporting so evident in the own-children estimates. This may have been due partly to use of an age-event chart of the type recommended by Takeshita for the collection of birth histories. In Korea, age reporting is known to be quite accurate, and the impact of age misreporting on the estimated fertility trends seems to be minimal. It likewise appears that in Dominican Republic and Syria age misreporting does not seriously distort the fertility estimates, although the age data are not as free from misreporting as in the Korean case.

None of the countries examined show much indication of a bunching of births in the birth histories in the vicinity of five to ten years before the survey; fertility ten to fourteen years before the survey tends to be about as high or higher than fertility five to ten years before the survey. Moreover, in at least one case, Pakistan, fertility during the five years immediately preceding the survey seems implausibly low, probably due to a pattern of age exaggeration stemming from upward rounding of children's ages. This mechanism probably operates in Indonesia as well, although independent evidence indicating a rapid rise in contraceptive use suggests that part of the indicated fertility decline in Indonesia is real. On the whole, Potter's hypothesis about misplacement of events, which assumes bunching of births five to ten years before the survey and accurate reporting of births during the first five years or so immediately preceding the survey, does not receive much support from these data. This finding reinforces previous work by Blacker and Brass (1979), who found evidence that recent dates of birth obtained from birth histories often tend to be pushed backward from rather than toward the survey date.

Overall, the data suggest that age misreporting is not an insuperable obstacle to collecting birth histories that yield reasonably accurate estimates of fertility trends. In this regard, it would be especially interesting and potentially useful to study in more detail the procedures by which the Nepal survey achieved such unusual accuracy in its birth histories despite severe age misreporting problems evident in the estimates based on own children. In half of the WFS surveys examined here, however, patterns of age misreporting are clearly reflected not only in fertility trends estimated from own children but also in trends estimated from birth histories.

In most cases, the agreement between the fertility estimates derived alternatively from own children and birth histories is impressive. Although this agreement may sometimes reflect common sources of error, the results suggest that household surveys are often adequate for estimating fertility levels and trends.

APPENDIX TABLE 1. Age-specific birth rates and values of CFR(35) estimated alternatively from birth histories and own children

	ASBR				
	15—19	20—24	25—29	30—34	CFR(35)
A. Nepal					
Birth histories					
1961	131	275	311	253	4845
1962	124	229	231	234	4095
1963	143	264	291	250	4737
1964	141	272	297	233	4714
1965	124	298	275	261	4792
1966	155	252	322	272	4998
1967	124	255	289	237	4527
1968	142	282	299	243	4827
1969	144	288	277	238	4739
1970	123	288	301	234	4732
1971	153	302	303	255	5067
1972	120	261	288	228	4487
1973	134	294	283	231	4706
1974	118	286	288	236	4644
1975	129	304	294	269	4978
Own children					
1961	110	271	297	228	4526
1962	109	203	214	210	3682
1963	192	323	370	277	5807
1964	121	221	217	225	3918
1965	185	322	357	303	5834
1966	116	245	223	167	3755
1967	161	277	306	294	5186
1968	142	310	298	235	4924
1969	133	274	288	239	4668
1970	170	306	317	272	5324
1971	137	285	276	229	4636
1972	117	254	265	232	4338
1973	110	241	263	202	4084
1974	91	263	245	218	4086
1975	94	255	262	226	4188

APPENDIX TABLE 1. *(continued)*

| | ASBR | | | | |
	15—19	20—24	25—29	30—34	CFR(35)
B. Pakistan					
Birth histories					
1961	171	292	314	238	5072
1962	176	295	298	283	5264
1963	174	318	370	300	5811
1964	144	292	296	258	4954
1965	192	316	351	325	5916
1966	154	325	321	272	5359
1967	158	309	339	274	5400
1968	166	320	330	308	5615
1969	184	324	312	297	5589
1970	144	321	345	290	5498
1971	171	276	342	253	5208
1972	140	306	357	294	5484
1973	122	270	278	249	4600
1974	130	248	284	239	4500
1975	132	294	328	262	5080
Own children					
1961	144	293	321	277	5174
1962	144	308	297	255	5022
1963	198	373	391	345	6536
1964	127	300	255	228	4549
1965	200	371	409	379	6794
1966	122	298	307	228	4776
1967	159	332	374	313	5894
1968	153	341	350	336	5898
1969	154	298	339	296	5434
1970	150	330	377	310	5835
1971	134	268	315	263	4897
1972	129	276	364	278	5233
1973	126	274	293	237	4650
1974	102	218	224	227	3860
1975	104	246	278	250	4392

APPENDIX TABLE 1. *(continued)*

| | ASBR | | | | CFR(35) |
	15—19	20—24	25—29	30—34	
C. Sri Lanka					
Birth histories					
1961	111	259	264	256	4455
1962	101	256	305	210	4358
1963	101	234	305	258	4488
1964	89	216	273	211	3944
1965	83	258	271	252	4318
1966	73	202	281	217	3864
1967	71	219	258	223	3852
1968	74	174	258	222	3640
1969	72	187	230	223	3562
1970	60	182	281	236	3800
1971	66	185	227	189	3337
1972	47	166	250	186	3238
1973	44	152	215	205	3076
1974	37	163	166	152	2586
1975	39	157	225	185	3028
Own children					
1961	107	261	248	247	4318
1962	96	259	284	234	4368
1963	96	264	317	280	4788
1964	86	200	268	217	3850
1965	86	234	280	278	4393
1966	67	194	251	213	3622
1967	63	215	255	226	3794
1968	73	172	262	221	3645
1969	60	170	218	211	3294
1970	53	175	264	230	3610
1971	60	170	204	185	3094
1972	40	150	226	195	3061
1973	37	142	200	192	2860
1974	29	139	145	138	2258
1975	29	132	186	167	2566

APPENDIX TABLE 1. *(continued)*

	ASBR				
	15—19	20—24	25—29	30—34	CFR(35)
D. Dominican Republic					
Birth histories					
1960	126	346	336	277	5422
1961	153	334	356	246	5443
1962	173	379	317	303	5862
1963	169	353	403	300	6126
1964	170	366	340	285	5803
1965	130	328	360	296	5572
1966	152	314	308	277	5258
1967	120	327	345	289	5402
1968	108	274	324	273	4896
1969	87	288	320	259	4768
1970	90	283	297	269	4696
1971	74	246	269	248	4184
1972	59	241	251	221	3864
1973	42	208	227	197	3372
1974	24	199	214	202	3192
Own children					
1960	166	344	340	299	5742
1961	165	325	334	266	5452
1962	160	362	356	323	6004
1963	169	308	320	285	5412
1964	180	370	358	278	5925
1965	146	309	335	251	5200
1966	152	307	345	297	5508
1967	142	340	370	294	5732
1968	127	291	301	275	4967
1969	109	259	309	261	4693
1970	116	280	294	280	4854
1971	108	241	289	253	4451
1972	109	263	259	211	4212
1973	100	225	231	198	3773
1974	105	230	229	183	3735

APPENDIX TABLE 1. *(continued)*

	ASBR				
	15—19	20—24	25—29	30—34	CFR(35)
E. Korea					
Birth histories					
1960	24	267	330	282	4514
1961	17	242	338	289	4428
1962	13	230	337	261	4204
1963	15	213	353	263	4216
1964	12	221	298	239	3852
1965	21	188	304	229	3712
1966	12	204	307	222	3730
1967	17	192	305	194	3540
1968	15	184	353	234	3932
1969	14	181	329	205	3642
1970	18	190	338	208	3767
1971	18	213	333	212	3882
1972	14	210	307	206	3680
1973	12	184	320	194	3552
1974	19	188	301	158	3330
Own children					
1960	27	258	313	282	4400
1961	20	236	313	249	4090
1962	19	202	308	266	3975
1963	17	208	345	260	4150
1964	12	208	293	205	3590
1965	22	188	305	221	3680
1966	13	201	311	219	3720
1967	18	183	304	186	3455
1968	17	180	330	230	3785
1969	17	192	332	216	3785
1970	20	178	343	199	3700
1971	17	217	331	223	3940
1972	13	200	304	216	3665
1973	14	179	325	200	3590
1974	17	183	281	147	3140

34

APPENDIX TABLE 1. *(continued)*

| | ASBR | | | | CFR(35) |
	15—19	20—24	25—29	30—34	
F. Syria					
Birth histories					
1964	143	332	378	356	6048
1965	141	323	353	385	6006
1966	166	373	391	350	6402
1967	145	321	377	307	5749
1968	148	334	369	364	6071
1969	145	319	365	360	5942
1970	121	328	351	303	5513
1971	136	313	340	326	5573
1972	118	305	347	302	5356
1973	108	305	362	317	5468
1974	139	281	342	325	5430
1975	135	311	310	310	5327
1976	123	294	344	346	5536
1977	113	298	362	274	5234
1978	110	296	328	303	5188
Own children					
1964	163	344	348	345	5999
1965	169	339	359	352	6096
1966	177	352	400	335	6319
1967	151	340	340	324	5774
1968	167	347	416	356	6428
1969	135	304	333	308	5396
1970	136	329	370	323	5786
1971	133	310	348	289	5400
1972	138	314	348	326	5630
1973	119	291	360	318	5440
1974	120	294	343	316	5364
1975	127	293	317	319	5280
1976	117	290	318	289	5074
1977	97	254	297	262	4551
1978	95	268	330	295	4936

APPENDIX TABLE 1. *(continued)*

	ASBR				
	15—19	20—24	25—29	30—34	CFR(35)
G. Indonesia					
Birth histories					
1961	191	278	249	203	4606
1962	146	234	227	183	3949
1963	179	285	258	218	4703
1964	136	243	231	200	4048
1965	193	288	276	232	4946
1966	118	247	246	211	4107
1967	161	251	244	219	4374
1968	149	268	264	206	4429
1969	168	258	262	196	4422
1970	142	270	227	207	4228
1971	142	274	265	208	4446
1972	132	268	237	195	4156
1973	114	231	213	146	3522
1974	111	201	208	122	3210
1975	125	272	208	164	3849
Own children					
1961	154	238	237	208	4188
1962	135	235	229	179	3885
1963	166	281	268	230	4722
1964	138	223	209	184	3767
1965	170	308	314	242	5170
1966	106	240	218	203	3836
1967	159	273	262	248	4710
1968	168	289	287	208	4760
1969	150	264	248	202	4320
1970	142	281	278	222	4615
1971	141	306	289	231	4830
1972	128	272	254	210	4320
1973	117	240	220	154	3654
1974	107	218	192	120	3184
1975	121	232	201	153	3539

APPENDIX TABLE 1. *(continued)*

	ASBR				
	15—19	20—24	25—29	30—34	CFR(35)
H. Kenya					
Birth histories					
1963	240	385	419	357	7008
1964	206	392	343	347	6436
1965	199	369	371	377	6578
1966	196	338	342	312	5940
1967	204	394	339	359	6478
1968	187	338	358	298	5904
1969	214	367	366	389	6680
1970	182	350	385	310	6130
1971	195	346	355	323	6093
1972	181	352	358	323	6066
1973	169	327	358	333	5938
1974	177	361	336	282	5786
1975	150	325	347	315	5683
1976	121	296	349	284	5246
1977	127	334	360	286	5536
Own children					
1963	262	388	392	345	6938
1964	206	374	363	326	6348
1965	204	452	368	361	6924
1966	172	311	359	274	5576
1967	222	411	350	284	6334
1968	150	384	338	358	6148
1969	193	377	392	307	6342
1970	178	341	368	329	6082
1971	182	329	321	277	5547
1972	156	313	368	304	5704
1973	141	328	337	316	5614
1974	161	333	348	279	5608
1975	154	310	327	316	5536
1976	132	286	321	267	5036
1977	155	284	308	259	5028

REFERENCES

Afzal, M.

1974   *The Population of Pakistan.* CICRED Monograph Series. Islamabad: Pakistan Institute of Development Economics.

Blacker, J., and W. Brass

1979   Experience of retrospective demographic enquiries to determine vital rates. In *The Recall Method in Social Surveys,* eds. L. Moss and H. Goldstein. London: University of London Institute of Education.

Brass, W.

1975   *Methods for Estimating Fertility and Mortality from Limited and Defective Data.* Chapel Hill: Laboratories for Population Statistics, University of North Carolina.

Chidambaram, V.C., and Z.A. Sathar

Forth-   *Age and Date Reporting.* Comparative Studies Series. London:
coming   World Fertility Survey.

Cho, L.J.

1973   The own-children approach to fertility estimation: an elaboration. In Vol. 2, *International Population Conference, Liège 1973,* 263–78. Liège: International Union for the Scientific Study of Population.

Coale, A.J., and P. Demeny

1966   *Regional Model Life Tables and Stable Populations.* Princeton: Princeton University Press.

Goldman, N., A.J. Coale, and M. Weinstein

1979   *The Quality of Data in the Nepal Fertility Survey.* World Fertility Survey Scientific Reports, No. 6. London: International Statistical Institute.

Guzman, J.M.

1980   *Evaluation of the Dominican Republic National Fertility Survey 1975.* Scientific Reports No. 14. London: World Fertility Survey.

Henin, R.A., A. Korten, and L.H. Werner

1982   *Evaluation of Birth Histories: A Case Study of Kenya.* Scientific Reports No. 36. London: World Fertility Survey.

Hobcraft, J., and G. Rodriguez

1982   *The Analysis of Repeat Fertility Surveys: Examples from Dominican Republic.* Scientific Reports No. 29. London: World Fertility Survey.

Jamai, H., and S. Singh

1984   Question design for measurement of selected demographic events. Paper presented at the World Fertility Survey Symposium, London, 24–27 April.

Little, R.J.A.

1982   *Sampling Errors of Fertility Rates from the WFS.* WFS Technical Bulletin No. 10. London: World Fertility Survey.

Potter, J.E.

1977   Problems in using birth-history analysis to estimate trends in fertility. *Population Studies* 31:335–64.

Ratnayake, K., R.D. Retherford, and S. Sivasubramaniam

1984   *Fertility Estimates for Sri Lanka Derived from the 1981 Census.* Colombo: Aitken Spence and Co.

Retherford, R.D.

1978   Single-year computational procedures used in the own-children method of fertility estimation. *Asian and Pacific Census Forum* 4(3):5–8.

Retherford, R.D., Aphichat Chamratrithirong, and Anuri Wanglee

1980   The impact of alternative mortality assumptions on own-children estimates of fertility for Thailand. *Asian and Pacific Census Forum* 6(3):5–8.

Retherford, R.D., and L.J. Cho

1978   Age-parity-specific birth rates and birth probabilities from census or survey data on own children. *Population Studies* 32:567–81.

Retherford, R.D., L.J. Cho, and N.I. Kim

1983   Estimates of current fertility derived from the 1980 census of the Republic of Korea. *Asian and Pacific Census Forum* 9(3):12–15.

Retherford, R.D., and M. Mirza

1982   Evidence of age exaggeration in demographic estimates for Pakistan. *Population Studies* 36:257–70.

Sri Lanka Department of Census and Statistics

1978   *Life Tables 1970–72: Sri Lanka.* Colombo: Department of Census and Statistics.

Supraptilah, B.

1982   *Evaluation of the Indonesian Fertility Survey 1976.* Scientific Reports No. 38. London: World Fertility Survey.